Sphincter of Oddi Dysfunction

A Beginner's 3-Step Guide to Managing SOD Through Diet, With Sample Curated Recipes

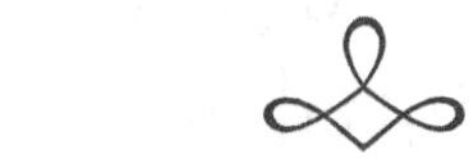

PATRICK MARSHWELL

Disclaimer

By reading this disclaimer, you are accepting the terms of the disclaimer in full. If you disagree with this disclaimer, please do not use this website.

All of the content within this website is provided for informational and educational purposes only, and should not be accepted as independent medical or other professional advice. The author of these articles is not a doctor, physician, nurse, mental health provider, or registered nutritionist/dietician. Therefore, using and reading any of the content on this website does not establish any form of a physician-patient relationship.

Always consult with a physician or another qualified health provider with any issues or questions you might have regarding any sort of medical condition. Do not ever disregard any qualified professional medical advice or delay seeking that advice because of anything you have read in this guide. The information in this guide is not intended to be any sort of medical advice and should not be used in lieu of any medical advice by a licensed and qualified medical professional.

The information on this website has been compiled from a variety of known sources. However, the author cannot attest to or guarantee the accuracy of each source and thus should not be held liable for any errors or omissions.

Introduction

The liver and pancreas are two organs that work together to produce digestive enzymes. These enzymes travel through a duct called the biliary system and are released into the small intestine to help with the digestion of food.

The sphincter of Oddi is a muscle located at the junction of the biliary system and the small intestine. It acts as a valve, opening to release enzymes into the small intestine and closing to prevent them from flowing back into the biliary system.

Sphincter of Oddi dysfunction (SOD) occurs when this muscle does not function properly. SOD can lead to abdominal pain, bloating, and diarrhea. It can also cause liver damage and pancreatitis.

Treatment for SOD typically involves medications to relax the sphincter of Oddi's muscle. In some cases, surgery may be necessary to remove the affected portion of the muscle.

Diet and lifestyle changes can also help to manage symptoms of SOD. avoiding triggers, such as fatty foods, alcohol, and caffeine; eating smaller meals more frequently, and managing stress can all help to reduce the frequency and severity of SOD symptoms.

In this beginner's guide, we'll discuss the following subtopics in detail:

- What are the two types of the sphincter of Oddi dysfunction?
- What causes the sphincter of Oddi dysfunction?
- What are the symptoms of SOD?
- Who is at risk for SOD?
- How is SOD diagnosed?
- What are the treatments for SOD?
- Managing SOD symptoms through lifestyle changes.
- Managing SOD through dietary changes.

If you or someone you know wants to know more about SOD, then this beginner's guide is for you. Read on to learn everything you need to know about this condition.

Table of Contents

WHAT ARE THE TWO TYPES OF THE SPHINCTER OF ODDI DYSFUNCTION?

There are two main types of the sphincter of Oddi dysfunction, including biliary dyskinesia, sphincter of Oddi stenosis, and pancreaticobiliary maljunction.

Biliary dyskinesia: Biliary dyskinesia is a relatively rare disorder that occurs when the sphincter of Oddi, a muscle that controls the flow of digestive juices from the liver, doesn't function properly. This can cause the juices to back up in the bile ducts, resulting in pain, nausea, and vomiting. In some cases, the condition can also lead to jaundice (yellowing of the skin and eyes) and itching. While the exact cause of biliary dyskinesia is unknown, it's thought to be associated with certain medical conditions, such as gallstones or pancreatitis.

Sphincter of Oddi stenosis: Sphincter of Oddi stenosis (SOS), also known as papillary stenosis, is a narrowing of the Sphincter of Oddi (SO), a muscle that controls the flow of bile and pancreatic juices into the small intestine. This condition can lead to pain, jaundice (yellowing of the skin and eyes), and pancreatitis. SOS occurs when the SO muscle contracts too strongly or goes into spasm, which narrows or blocks the opening through which bile and pancreatic juice pass.

While all two types of the sphincter of Oddi dysfunction can be painful and potentially dangerous, prompt diagnosis and treatment are essential for maintaining good health.

WHAT CAUSES THE SPHINCTER OF ODDI DYSFUNCTION?

There are several possible causes of Sphincter of Oddi dysfunction, including gallstones, inflammation of the Sphincter of Oddi, pancreatitis, or damage to the Sphincter of Oddi from surgery.

Gallstone: Gallstones are one of the most common causes of sphincter of Oddi dysfunction. Gallstones are small, hard deposits that form in the gallbladder. They can block the flow of bile and pancreatic juices, causing them to back up and leading to pain. In some cases, surgery may be necessary to remove the gallstones and relieve the pain.

Inflammation: Sphincter of Oddi dysfunction (SOD) is a condition that can be caused by inflammation of the Sphincter of Oddi. When the Sphincter of Oddi is inflamed, it can cause a build-up of these fluids, which can in turn lead to pain, nausea, and vomiting. SOD is often caused by a viral infection or autoimmune disease.

Overuse of pain medications: SOD is thought to be caused by overuse of pain medications like opioids. Opioids increase pressure in the biliary system, which can lead to SOD.

In addition, opioids can damage the nerves that control the sphincter of Oddi, causing it to spasm.

Pancreatitis: Pancreatitis can lead to the sphincter of Oddi dysfunction. Pancreatitis is an inflammation of the pancreas, which is a large gland behind the stomach that releases enzymes that help with digestion. It can be caused by drinking too much alcohol, certain medications, or certain medical conditions.

Surgery: When surgery is performed on the bile duct, gallbladder, or pancreas, the Sphincter of Oddi can be damaged, causing it to malfunction. In some cases, SOD may also be caused by scarring from previous surgery. While the exact incidence of SOD after surgery is unknown, it is thought to be a relatively rare complication. However, it is important to be aware of the potential risks before undergoing any type of surgery.

WHAT ARE THE SYMPTOMS OF SPHINCTER OF ODDI DYSFUNCTION?

If you encounter any of the following symptoms, you should make an appointment to see a medical professional as soon as possible since they may be an indication of SOD:

Severe abdominal pain that typically comes in waves: One of the symptoms of Sphincter of Oddi Dysfunction is severe stomach discomfort, which often comes and goes in waves. The muscle that controls the opening and closure of the sphincter may be at fault for the pain you are experiencing.

This inhibits bile and pancreatic secretions from draining correctly, which leads to their building up and leaking back into the pancreas, which in turn causes inflammation in the pancreas. Sphincter of Oddi contractions is the root cause of the waves of agony that patients experience. Even while the pain might be rather acute at times, it is not normally consistent.

Nausea and vomiting: Sphincter of Oddi Dysfunction is characterized by several symptoms, the most prevalent of which are nausea and vomiting (SOD). A muscle known as the sphincter of Oddi, which is situated at the point where the bile duct and the pancreatic duct meet, can become afflicted with a condition known as SOD.

The sphincter of Oddi is a valve that controls the passage of bile and pancreatic fluids into the small intestine. It does this by acting as a barrier. These digestive fluids can back up when the sphincter of Oddi is not working properly, which can cause symptoms such as nausea, vomiting, stomach discomfort, and bloating.

Pain that gets worse after eating fatty foods: After consuming a meal that is particularly high in fat, it is not unusual to suffer some discomfort in the stomach region. However, if this pain is severe and grows worse after eating fatty meals, it may be a sign of Sphincter of Oddi Dysfunction. This may be diagnosed by observing whether or not the discomfort gets worse after eating fatty foods (SOD).

Jaundice (yellowing of the skin and eyes): Sphincter of Oddi Dysfunction is characterized by several symptoms, the most prominent of which is jaundice, sometimes known as a yellowing of the skin. This is because the Sphincter of Oddi is a valve that regulates the passage of bile from the liver to the small intestine. As a result, this phenomenon takes place. Jaundice can develop when this valve does not operate as it should, which can allow bile to accumulate in the liver.

Diarrhea: Sphincter of Oddi Dysfunction is also frequently accompanied by the symptom of diarrhea. SOD has been linked to an accumulation of bile and pancreatic secretions, which has the potential to result in diarrhea. SOD causes diarrhea that is frequently watery and may be accompanied by stomach discomfort, cramps, bloating, and gas.

Clay-colored stools: Sphincter of Oddi Dysfunction can be identified by feces that have a clay-like consistency. Clay-colored feces are a result of bile being present in the stool, which might be an indication that the Sphincter of Oddi is not working as it should. If you have stools that are the color of clay, you should make an appointment with your primary care physician as soon as possible to rule out any other potential reasons, such as gallstones or pancreatitis.

Dark urine: A further sign of Sphincter of Oddi Dysfunction is urine that is dark in color. When the sphincter of Oddi does not work as it should, bile can accumulate in the liver, which can result in urine that is discolored. If your urine is black, you should make an appointment with your doctor as soon as possible so that other potential reasons may be ruled out.

There are therapies available that, even though SOD is sometimes difficult to diagnose, can help to improve both symptoms and quality of life. If you are concerned that you may have SOD, you should discuss being tested with your primary care physician.

WHO IS AT RISK FOR SOD?

SOD may happen to anybody, although it is significantly more frequent in women and persons who have had surgery on their pancreas or bile duct in the past. SOD is also more likely to develop in persons who have specific medical disorders, such as inflammatory bowel disease or gallstones. These factors make SOD more likely to arise.

Age and Gender: The chance of having a Sphincter of Oddi Dysfunction (SOD) can be influenced by several different variables, including gender. SOD strikes persons between the ages of 20 and 50 years old the majority of the time, and it is more prevalent in girls than in males.

There are a few different hypotheses to explain this phenomenon, even if the causes behind it are not completely known. One idea proposes that hormones are involved in the process of SOD formation in the body. The levels of estrogen and progesterone in a woman's body alter throughout her lifetime, and these variations can affect how the sphincter of Oddi works.

People who have had surgery on the bile duct or pancreas: Scarring from prior surgery, inflammation, or injury to the nerves that regulate the sphincter muscle can also induce spasms of the esophageal diaphragm (SOD). SOD is more likely to occur in patients who have previously undergone surgery on either the bile duct or the pancreas.

People with certain medical conditions: Sphincter of Oddi Dysfunction is more likely to occur in patients who have a history of certain medical disorders. Gallstones, liver disease, pancreatitis, and Crohn's disease are some of the disorders that fall under this category. Additionally at risk are individuals who have already had their gallbladders removed.

You must consult a medical professional if you have any reason to believe that you may be at risk of having SOD. They will be able to explain the variables that put you at risk and give suggestions for the treatment or prevention of the condition.

HOW IS SPHINCTER OF ODDI DYSFUNCTION DIAGNOSED?

Sphincter of Oddi Dysfunction, often known as SOD, is a medical condition that has a record for being difficult to diagnose. A muscle known as the sphincter of Oddi can be found at the point where the small and large intestines join together. Endoscopic retrograde cholangiopancreatography (ERCP), magnetic resonance cholangiopancreatography (MRCP), and liver function tests are the most common tests that physicians would order while attempting to identify SOD in a patient. There are circumstances in which a laparoscopic exploration could also be required.

Endoscopic retrograde cholangiopancreatography (ERCP): Endoscopic retrograde cholangiopancreatography (ERCP) is a diagnostic technique that makes use of an endoscope to examine the bile and pancreatic channels. A contrast dye is injected into the biliary tree as well as the pancreatic duct while the treatment is being performed.

The dye gives the physician the ability to see any abnormalities or obstructions that may be present in the ducts. ERCP can also be used to treat SOD. This treatment involves relaxing the sphincter of Oddi, which enables a more unrestricted flow of bile.

Magnetic resonance cholangiopancreatography (MRCP): Magnetic resonance computed cholangiopancreatography, or MRCP, is a non-invasive imaging technique that employs MRI to examine the biliary tree and pancreatic duct. A diagnosis of SOD can be made with the use of MRCP by locating any blockages or abnormalities in the ducts.

Liver function tests: The levels of enzymes in the liver may be measured through blood tests that are referred to as liver function tests (LFTs). Proteins known as enzymes are generated by the liver to assist with a variety of chemical processes that take place throughout the body. The levels of enzymes in the blood will be high if the liver is not performing its functions as it should. Tests that evaluate liver function can be utilized to detect SOD by determining whether or not the liver has been damaged.

Laparoscopic exploration: Laparoscopic exploration could be required to diagnose SOD in certain patients, depending on the circumstances. During this technique, a tiny camera is introduced into the belly by making a very small incision in the skin. The biliary tree and pancreatic duct may both be visualized with the use of the camera. Laparoscopic exploration may be used to diagnose SOD by locating any blockages or anomalies in the ducts. This can be done through the process of detecting the obstructions.

If you have any reason to suspect that you may be suffering from a sphincter of Oddi dysfunction, you must discuss your concerns with a medical professional as soon as possible. They will be able to make a diagnosis after doing the necessary tests that they have ordered.

WHAT ARE THE TREATMENTS FOR THE SPHINCTER OF ODDI DYSFUNCTION?

Medical and surgical procedures are the two primary types of therapy options available for dysfunction of the sphincter of Oddi.

The majority of medical therapies include the administration of medication in one of two ways: either to relax the muscle that controls the sphincter or to promote the flow of bile down the duct. When all other therapy options have been exhausted, one may then contemplate surgical intervention.

Anti-spasm medicines: Medications that inhibit spasms are frequently the first line of defense in treating the condition. These medications work to relax the muscle in the sphincter, which in turn helps to ease discomfort.

Sphincterotomy: A sphincterotomy is an option that may be suggested if anti-spasm medications are ineffective or if the patient's symptoms are particularly severe. Sphincterotomy is a surgical operation that involves making an incision in the sphincter muscle. This helps to reduce discomfort and improves the muscle's ability to perform its function.

A sphincterotomy is a therapy that is both effective and safe for SOD. However, just like every other type of surgical operation, this one comes with its fair share of potential complications. Before deciding whether or not sphincterotomy is the correct choice for you, you and your physician should talk about the dangers involved.

Balloon dilation and endoscopic ultrasonography-guided biliary drainage are two examples of less invasive techniques that have the potential to be useful treatment options.

Balloon Dilation: Balloon dilation is a minimally invasive treatment that includes inserting a balloon into the bile duct and then inflating the balloon to widen the channel. Balloon dilation is also known as endoscopic balloon dilation. This reduces the amount of pressure placed on the sphincter muscle and makes it possible for bile to flow more freely.

Endoscopic Ultrasonography-Guided Biliary Drainage: Endoscopic Ultrasonography-Guided Biliary Drainage is a minimally invasive treatment that utilizes ultrasound to guide a drainage tube into the bile duct. This operation is sometimes referred to as EUGD. The drainage tube removes any extra bile that may have built up in the duct so that it may be used again.

Pancreatectomy: In very extreme circumstances, a complete pancreatectomy can be required. The surgical procedure known as a pancreatectomy removes all or part of a person's

14

pancreas. However, due to the inherent dangers, this strategy is almost always reserved for use as a last resort.

Collaborating with a gastroenterologist to devise a treatment strategy that is adapted to your specific requirements to treat Sphincter of Oddi Dysfunction is the most effective method for treating this condition.

MANAGING SYMPTOMS OF SOD THROUGH NATURAL METHODS

There is currently no known cure for sphincter of Oddi dysfunction; however, there are natural treatments that may be utilized to assist in the management of SOD-related symptoms.

Dietary changes: Alterations to one's diet will prove to be of more assistance in the long-term management of SOD symptoms. It is critical to maintaining a diet of several, more frequent, smaller meals throughout the day. The symptoms of stomach discomfort and bloating will be alleviated as a result of this action. You must stay away from meals that bring on your symptoms. Keeping a food journal might help determine what causes an episode.

Stress management: Because stress can make symptoms of SOD worse, you must find methods to relax and cut down on the amount of stress in your life. Yoga, meditation, and other practices like deep breathing exercises are examples of stress management methods that may be of some use.

Acupuncture: A kind of traditional Chinese medicine known as acupuncture involves putting very thin needles into the body at strategic spots. Acupuncture is also known as needling. It is believed that this will accelerate the flow of energy, also known as qi, and facilitate healing. It is possible to manage pain with acupuncture, particularly the sort of abdominal pain that is linked with SOD.

If you are thinking about attempting acupuncture for SOD, it is essential that you first have a conversation with a trained professional in the field. When conducted by a competent expert, acupuncture is generally regarded as safe; nonetheless, there are certain hazards associated with the procedure. These include discomfort at the location of the needle, bruising, and bleeding at the site. Before beginning therapy, you should make it a point to share any concerns that you have with your practitioner.

Magnesium supplements: Magnesium supplementation is one natural treatment option that has the potential to help alleviate symptoms of SOD. Magnesium is a mineral that is involved in more than 300 different metabolic events that take place in the body. Studies have indicated that it can assist to lessen the number of spasms that occur in the intestines, and it is involved in the process of relaxing muscles.

In addition to this, magnesium possesses anti-inflammatory characteristics, which make it useful in assisting in the reduction of inflammation in the digestive tract. Have a discussion with your primary care provider to determine whether or not taking magnesium in supplement form is appropriate for you.

Lavender oil: It has been demonstrated that the essential oil of lavender helps relax smooth muscle, which can aid in the reduction of abdominal discomfort linked with SOD. In addition, lavender oil possesses characteristics that assist reduce inflammation and nausea, both of which are common SOD symptoms that can be alleviated by using the oil.

A single drop of 100% pure lavender essential oil can be added to a glass of water to create a relaxing atmosphere. Drink the water in little, spaced-out sips.

Castor oil pack: Castor oil packs are one form of natural therapy that is effective for SOD. Castor oil is massaged into a piece of flannel or cloth, which is then put over the patient's abdomen, as part of this treatment modality. After that, the flannel is wrapped in a heating pad or a hot water bottle, and the treatment is continued for thirty to sixty minutes.

This procedure can be carried out several times every week. Castor oil packs have been shown to assist enhance the quality of life for certain individuals by reducing the severity of their symptoms.

Chamomile tea: The Chamomile plant is used to make a variety of herbal teas, including the well-known Chamomile tea. Tea made from chamomile flowers has a long history of usage as a home treatment for a range of conditions, including gastrointestinal distress and indigestion.

Compounds included in chamomile tea have been shown to have the potential to relax the smooth muscle lining of the digestive system. This, in turn, makes it simpler for the contents of the stomach to move through the digestive tract. Additionally, there is some evidence that drinking chamomile tea might help decrease inflammation in the digestive tract.

If you are experiencing difficulties associated with SOD, it is essential to see your physician on the therapies that could be most appropriate for you. However, in addition to conventional treatment, trying out certain alternative therapies could be beneficial to your overall quality of life.

MANAGING SOD THROUGH DIET

It might be challenging to make dietary adjustments to treat the sphincter of Oddi dysfunction. Consuming foods that are not only nourishing to your body but also easy on your digestive system is an important part of a healthy lifestyle. Consuming a series of lighter meals spread throughout the day is an effective strategy for accomplishing this goal.

However, you should avoid fasting for an extended period since this may make your symptoms much more severe. In a perfect world, you would break up your day with a few light meals and some nutritious snacks every few hours. Because of this, you will be able to obtain the necessary nourishment without placing an excessive amount of effort on your digestive system.

Foods to avoid

Fatty Foods: Fatty meals are not only difficult to digest but also have the potential to exacerbate SOD symptoms. Steer clear of fried meals, processed meats, dairy products with full fat, and any other items that are rich in fat.

Spicy Foods: Spicy meals have been linked to an increase in stomach discomfort and other SOD symptoms. If you like particularly hot foods, you should attempt to cut back on how much you eat of them or completely avoid them.

Caffeine: The symptoms of SOD, including stomach discomfort and diarrhea, might be made worse by caffeine use. Your use of caffeinated beverages like coffee, tea, and soda should be kept to a minimum if at all possible.

Alcohol: The symptoms of SOD, which might include stomach discomfort, nausea, and vomiting, can be brought on by drinking alcohol. If you want to consume alcohol, do so in moderation at all times.

Foods to eat

Probiotic-rich foods: Probiotics are living microorganisms that are beneficial to the health of your digestive tract. Consuming probiotic-rich foods like yogurt, kefir, sauerkraut, and kimchi can help to improve digestion and lessen symptoms of SOD. Other foods that include probiotics include kimchi.

Soluble fiber: A gel-like material is formed in the digestive tract by soluble fiber, which dissolves in water. This particular type of fiber can assist to add bulk to stools, which in turn makes them easier to pass. Oats, lentils, flaxseeds, and chia seeds are all excellent food choices that provide soluble fiber in sufficient amounts.

Insoluble fiber: Insoluble fiber does not dissolve in water and cannot be digested by the body. This particular form of fiber makes feces bulkier, which in turn helps them travel through the digestive system more rapidly. Wheat bran, vegetables, and foods made with whole grains are all excellent sources of insoluble fiber.

Healthy fats: Olive oil, avocados, and almonds are all examples of foods that contain healthy fats that can help lessen the symptoms of SOD and encourage regular bowel movements.

Herbs and supplements

There are a few medicinal plants and dietary supplements that have shown some promise in alleviating the symptoms of SOD. However, before taking any herbs or supplements, it is essential to have a discussion with your primary care physician about the possibility of interactions with the prescriptions you are already taking.

Peppermint oil: Indigestion and other digestive issues are often treated with peppermint oil, which is a popular herbal medicine. The smooth muscular lining of the digestive system can be helped to relax by using peppermint oil, which contains substances that have this effect. This may help alleviate some of the symptoms of SOD, such as stomach discomfort and diarrhea.

Ginger: Ginger is a common plant that is used as a treatment for motion sickness and nausea. Ginger has been shown to have anti-inflammatory effects on the digestive tract as well as a relaxing effect on the smooth muscle that lines the digestive tract. This could help alleviate the symptoms of SOD.

Turmeric: Curcumin is a molecule that has potent anti-inflammatory properties, and turmeric, which is a spice, includes this substance. Curcumin is effective in relieving symptoms of SOD and reducing inflammation in the digestive tract.

Probiotics: Probiotics are living bacteria that are beneficial to the health of the digestive tract. It's possible that taking a probiotic pill might assist improve digestion and lessen the symptoms of SOD.

Elimination diet

Since you and everyone else are unique, you might need to try out a few various diets before settling on the one that gives you the greatest results. However, with some research and some experimentation, you should be able to discover a diet that not only helps lessen your symptoms but also makes it simpler for you to live with the sphincter of Oddi dysfunction that you have.

The Symptoms of Oddi symptoms may sometimes be traced back to certain foods, and one approach to narrow down the list is to go on an elimination diet. On the other hand, there is insufficient data to justify its utilization for this objective. As a result of this, it is essential to have a conversation with your primary care physician before making any modifications to your diet. If you do have dysfunction of the sphincter of Oddi, adopting an elimination diet may help reduce some of the symptoms you experience.

The purpose of an elimination diet is to rid your diet of foods that might potentially set off an allergic reaction, after which you will gradually reintroduce the foods one at a time. This gives you the ability to determine which meals could be causing your problems.

The elimination diet might be carried out in the following manner:

Step 1: Remove potential triggers from your diet

The first thing you should do is change your diet so that it excludes any possible triggers. If you believe that consuming hot foods makes your SOD symptoms worse, for instance, you should avoid eating spicy foods while you are in the elimination phase of the treatment.

There are a few distinct approaches to taking care of this matter. Following a pre-made elimination diet plan is one of the available options. Another choice is to design your elimination diet according to the symptoms and food sensitivities you have been experiencing.

Eliminating the most frequent triggers, such as meals that are hot and foods that are high in fat, is a good place to start if you are unsure of which foods may be causing your symptoms.

Step 2: Reintroduce foods one at a time

After you have removed all probable triggers from your diet, you will be able to slowly reintroduce foods back into your routine one by one. Begin by eliminating the meal that you believe has the smallest possibility of causing your symptoms.

For instance, if you have cut out very hot items as well as dairy products from your diet, you might want to begin by reintroducing dairy products.

Consume the food in question daily for three to five days before reintroducing it. You may presume that the meal is safe for you to eat if you do not have any sort of reaction to it within that period.

If you do experience a reaction, you must refrain from consuming the food in question and see a medical professional. They will be able to assist you in determining if the food is indeed the source of your symptoms or whether there may be another contributing factor.

Step 3: Identify your triggers

You should be able to determine which foods are causing your symptoms once you have reintroduced all of the possible triggers into your diet and done so in order from most likely to least likely.

If you find that you do not react when you eat dairy products but that you do experience symptoms after eating spicy foods, you may want to avoid eating spicy foods in the future. For example, if you find that you do not react when you eat dairy products but that you do experience symptoms after eating spicy foods.

If you are unsure as to whether a certain meal is causing your symptoms, you may always try eliminating that food from your diet once again and see if it makes a difference in how your symptoms are affected.

SAMPLE RECIPES

Kimchi Omelet

Ingredients:

- 1/4 cup and 2 tbsp. kimchi, chopped
- scallions, sliced thinly
- 2 eggs
- olive oil
- sea salt
- 2 tbsp. nori, sliced thinly

Instructions:

1. In a bowl, mix well the 1/4 cup of kimchi, scallion, and eggs.
2. Add olive oil to the pan.
3. Pour the egg mixture and let it cook.
4. Add sea salt to taste. Put 2 tbsp. of kimchi in the center.
5. Fold the omelet and place it on a plate.
6. Sprinkle nori and serve while hot.

Cucumber with Fennel and Creamy Avocado Dressing

Ingredients:

- 2 cups sliced cucumber
- 1/2 medium avocado, peeled and pit discarded
- 1/4 tsp. and a dash salt
- freshly ground black pepper, to taste
- 2 tbsp. fresh lemon juice
- 1 large fennel, outer layer removed
- 1 tbsp. finely chopped chives

Instructions:

1. In a large bowl, combine cucumber and fennel.
2. Toss with 1/4 tsp. of salt and pepper. Set aside.
3. In a food processor, combine avocado and lemon juice. Process until smooth for about 20 seconds.
4. Add the avocado mixture to the cucumber mixture. Combine thoroughly.
5. Add chives and a dash of salt.
6. Serve and enjoy at once.

Asian-Themed Macrobiotic Bowl

Ingredients:

- 2 cups cooked quinoa
- 4 carrots
- 1 package of smoked tofu
- 1 tbsp. nutritional yeast
- 2 tbsp. coconut aminos
- 4 tbsp. sunflower sprouts
- 2 tbsp. fermented vegetables
- 1 cup of shiitake mushrooms

- 1 avocado
- 2 tbsp. hemp seeds
- 2-3 cooked beets
- coconut oil cooking spray

Dressing:

- 2 tbsp. miso paste
- 1 tbsp. tahini
- 1 clove garlic, crushed
- 1 tbsp. olive oil
- 1/2 lime, juiced
- 3 tbsp. water

Instructions:

1. Roast the carrots in the oven at 400°F for 30-40 minutes.
2. Wash the vegetables, trim, and spray them with coconut oil.
3. Add them in the oven. When they are cooked, set aside till you are ready to assemble the Buddha bowl.
4. Make the dressing by combining all of the ingredients in a medium-size bowl. If the dressing appears lumpy, add more water.
5. To build the bowl, put the quinoa on the bottom and then arrange the vegetables on top.
6. Sprinkle the bowls with hemp seeds and drizzle the dressing over top.
7. Now serve and enjoy!

Broccoli-Kale with Avocado Toppings Rice Bowl

Ingredients:

- 1/2 avocado
- 2 cups kale
- 1 cup broccoli florets
- 1/2 cup cooked brown rice
- 1 tsp. plum vinegar
- 2 tsp. tamari
- sea salt, to taste

Instructions:

1. In a small pot, simmer broccoli florets, and kale in about 3 tbsp. of water. Cook for 2 minutes.
2. Add tamari, vinegar, and cooked brown rice. Stir to combine.
3. Transfer pot contents into a medium-sized bowl and top with sliced avocado; sprinkle a dash of sea salt to taste.
4. Serve immediately.

Avocado, Cucumber, and Tomato Salad

Ingredients:

- 1/4 cup extra-virgin olive oil
- 1 pc. lemon, juiced
- 1/4 tsp. cumin, ground
- salt, to taste
- freshly ground black pepper, to taste
- 3 medium avocados, cubed

- 1-pint cherry tomatoes, halved
- 1 small cucumber, sliced into half-moons
- 1/3 cup corn
- 2 tbsp. cilantro, chopped

Instructions:

1. Combine avocados, cilantro, corn, cucumber, jalapeño, and tomatoes in a large bowl.
2. In a separate small container, whisk together lemon juice, cumin, and oil to make the salad dressing.
3. Season the dressing with salt and pepper.
4. Toss the salad gently while adding the dressing.
5. Serve immediately.

Arugula and Mushroom Salad

Ingredients:

- 5 oz. arugula washed
- 1 lb. fresh mushrooms
- 1/4 tsp. shoyu
- 1/2 red onion
- 1 tbsp. olive oil
- 1 tbsp. mirin

For tofu cheese:

- 1/8 cup umeboshi vinegar
- 1/2 firm tofu

Instructions:

1. In a bowl, add the rinsed tofu. Crumble and pour in vinegar.
2. In a separate bowl add shoyu, red onions, salt, olive oil, and mirin. 3. Mix to combine.
3. Add in the arugula and toss to combine with the dressing.
4. Serve and enjoy.

Asian Zucchini Salad

Ingredients:

- 1 medium zucchini, sliced thinly into spirals
- 1/3 cup rice vinegar
- 3/4 cup avocado oil
- 1 cup sunflower seeds, shells removed
- 1 lb. cabbage, shredded
- 1 tsp. stevia drops
- 1 cup almonds, sliced

Instructions:

1. Cut the zucchini spirals into smaller parts. Set aside.
2. Put almonds, sunflower seeds, and cabbage in a large bowl. Combine the ingredients well.
3. Add zucchini to the mixture.
4. In a small bowl, mix vinegar, stevia, and oil using a whisk or fork.
5. Pour vinegar mixture all over the zucchini mixture. Toss well. Make sure everything is covered with the dressing.
6. Refrigerate for 2 hours before serving.

Asparagus and Greens Salad with Tahini and Poppy Seed Dressing

Ingredients:

- 10 to 12 asparagus stalks, washed well and sliced into ribbons
- 5 radishes, washed well, and sliced thinly
- 2 to 3 rainbow carrots, peeled and sliced thinly
- 1 handful wild spinach
- 1 small handful of microgreens, washed well
- 1 small handful of sunflower greens, washed well
- optional: few pieces of chive blossoms

For the dressing:

- 2 tbsp. tahini
- 1 tbsp. poppy seeds
- 1 tbsp. extra-virgin olive oil
- salt
- pepper

Instructions:

1. For the dressing, whisk ingredients together in a small bowl.
2. In a separate bowl, toss salad ingredients in the mixture.
3. Drizzle dressing on salad upon serving.

Mediterranean Vegetables

Ingredients:

- 16 oz. mixed frozen broccoli, carrots, and cauliflower
- 1 tbsp. drained capers
- 1 can diced tomatoes, basil, garlic, and oregano

Instructions:

1. Combine tomatoes, mixed vegetables, and drained capers in a microwave-safe bowl.
2. Cover with plastic wrap.
3. Bake for 6 to 8 minutes on high heat.
4. Stir halfway.
5. Serve and enjoy.

Mixed Vegetable Roast with Lemon Zest

Ingredients:

- 1-1/2 cups broccoli florets
- 1-1/2 cups cauliflower florets
- 3/4 cup red bell pepper, diced
- 3/4 cup zucchini, diced
- 2 thinly sliced cloves of garlic
- 2 tsp. lemon zest
- 1 tbsp. olive oil
- a pinch of salt
- 1 tsp. dried and crushed oregano

Instructions:

1. Preheat the oven to 425°F for 25 minutes.

2. Combine garlic and florets of broccoli and cauliflower in a baking pan.
3. Drizzle oil evenly over the vegetables. Season with salt and oregano.
4. Stir the vegetables to coat them evenly.
5. Place the pan inside the oven and roast for 10 minutes.
6. Add zucchini and bell pepper to the mix. Toss to combine.
7. Continue roasting for 10 to 15 minutes more until the vegetables turn light brown.
8. Drizzle lemon zest over vegetables and toss.
9. Serve and enjoy.

Roasted Okra and Smoked Paprika

Ingredients:

- 1/2 tsp. pepper
- 1/4 tsp. garlic powder
- 1-1/2 tsp. smoked paprika
- 3 lb. fresh okra pods
- 3/4 tsp. salt
- 3 tbsp. lemon juice
- 3 tbsp. olive oil

Instructions:

1. Preheat the oven to 400°F.
2. Toss together all ingredients.
3. Arrange them in a baking pan.
4. Roast okra until they are lightly browned and tender.
5. Serve and enjoy.

Quinoa Stuffed Peppers

Ingredients:

- 4 sweet bell peppers, halved vertically, with ribs and seeds removed
- 3/4 cup quinoa, well rinsed
- 15 oz. tomatoes, diced
- 4 cups basil leaves
- 10 oz. baby spinach
- 1 clove garlic, small
- 1/4 cup pistachios, unsalted
- 6 tbsp. grated parmesan cheese
- 3 tbsp. extra-virgin olive oil
- 3 tbsp. boiling water
- 1/4 tsp. kosher salt
- a pinch of black pepper, freshly ground

Instructions:

1. Combine the basil, garlic, parmesan cheese, olive oil, black pepper, and a pinch of salt in a food processor or blender.
2. Blend until the texture of the mixture appears finely chopped.
3. Stir in the boiling water.

To make the stuffed peppers:

1. Place the bell pepper halves with the side up on a lightly oiled baking sheet.

2. Roast in the oven using the high setting for about 10 minutes, or until they start to soften and have become slightly charred.
3. Remove the peppers from the oven. Set them aside.
4. In a medium pot, let the quinoa and tomatoes simmer in the vegetable broth for 10 minutes.
5. Stir in the baby spinach in small batches.
6. Scoop the quinoa-spinach mixture. Place them into the roasted peppers.
7. Drizzle the filled bell peppers with pesto sauce.
8. Garnish with pistachios on top upon serving.

Summary

A malfunction of the sphincter of Oddi, which is the gateway between the stomach and the small intestine, is referred to as the sphincter of Oddi dysfunction. There are two forms of SOD, referred to respectively as acute and chronic. Chronic SOD is a condition that lasts for a long period, in contrast to acute SOD, which manifests itself suddenly and for a shorter period. It is not known what causes the dysfunction of the sphincter of Oddi; however, it might be brought on by several different things, such as an infection, an accident, or surgery.

Pain in the upper abdomen, nausea, vomiting, and diarrhea are some of the symptoms that can be experienced when the sphincter of Oddi is dysfunctional. Those who have had surgery on the gallbladder or bile ducts, those who have had an infection in the pancreatic ducts, and those who have diabetes are all at an increased risk of developing sphincter of Oddi dysfunction.

The malfunction of the sphincter of Oddi can be identified using several different techniques, such as an ultrasound, CT scan, or MRI. The treatment for sphincter of Oddi dysfunction is contingent on the nature of the problem as well as its degree of severity. Medications, surgical procedures, and natural treatments including dietary and lifestyle adjustments are all potential treatment choices. It might be difficult to manage the symptoms of Oddi dysfunction, but with the appropriate therapy, the vast majority of patients can lead reasonably normal lives.

References

Crittenden, J. P., & Dattilo, J. B. (2022). Sphincter of oddi dysfunction. In StatPearls. StatPearls Publishing. http://www.ncbi.nlm.nih.gov/books/NBK557871/.

Jacky. (2020, June 17). Is there a natural treatment for sphincter of oddi dysfunction? https://www.nutroo.me/is-there-a-natural-treatment-for-sphincter-of-oddi-dysfunction/.

Natural remedies for sphincter of oddi dysfunction. (n.d.). Retrieved October 20, 2022, from https://www.earthclinic.com/cures/sphincter-of-oddi-dysfunction.html.

Sphincter of oddi dysfunction. (n.d.). Cleveland Clinic. Retrieved October 20, 2022, from https://my.clevelandclinic.org/health/diseases/14516-sphincter-of-oddi-dysfunction.

Sphincter of Oddi Dysfunction. Cedars-Sinai. https://www.cedars-sinai.org/health-library/diseases-and-conditions/s/sphincter-of-oddi-dysfunction.html.